THE PANCREATITIS HANDBOOK: AN EASY-TO-READ GUIDE

Tony Poltrona

Disclaimer

The information provided in this book is solely for informational purposes. It is not intended to provide medical advice, to diagnose, treat, cure, or prevent any diseases or medical conditions, and is not a substitute for professional medical advice and care.

This book is dedicated to my Aunt Teresa
who died in 1987 from pancreatic cancer.

Table of Contents

1. INTRODUCTION

Pancreatitis is inflammation of the pancreas. Pancreatitis can come on suddenly and with little or no warning. This is known as **acute pancreatitis**. When pancreatitis symptoms such as nausea and pain continue or return frequently, the condition is called *chronic pancreatitis*. Both forms of pancreatitis are serious and can lead to life-threatening complications such as internal bleeding, infection, and permanent damage to or death of pancreatic tissue.

This easy-to-read guide to Pancreatitis explores a wide range of topics including…
- Structure and function of the pancreas
- Definition and types of pancreatitis
- Symptoms of pancreatitis
- Causes of pancreatitis
- Diagnosing pancreatitis
- Complications of pancreatitis
- Treating pancreatitis
- Prognosis

The end of this book provides three additional sections:
- Resources—a list of books, websites, and other resources to which you can refer for additional information about pancreatitis
- Eating for Pancreatitis—a guide to foods and suggested meal plans for keeping your pancreatitis at bay
- Recipes for Pancreatitis—a selection of low-fat or non-fat recipes that have been adapted for dealing with pancreatitis while not sacrificing too much flavor and taste

This book was written as an easy-to-read reference and guide for people who suffer from or have been diagnosed with pancreatitis.

The information provided in this guidebook is based on intensive and extensive reading about pancreatitis using a number of different sources. This information has been boiled down to be succinct and easily understandable even for someone without any health or medical-related knowledge.

Paragraphs and sentences have intentionally been kept short and easy to understand. This book also presents a good amount of information in the form of lists, tables, and diagrams because, as they say, a picture is worth a thousand words!

2. WHAT IS A PANCREAS?

2.1 What a Strange Word

The word **pancreas** (pronounced **pan**-*kree-us*) is derived from the Greek word *pánkreas*, which means "sweetbread", "flesh", or "meat."

In order to understand pancreatitis, it is helpful to understand the basic structure and functions of the pancreas.

2.2 Size, Shape, and Color

The pancreas is a long, slender gland with a thick head and a body that tapers to a tail. It is yellowish in color, about six to eight inches long, and about one-and-a-half inches thick.

The pancreas is "divided" into four segments or sections (see figure 1):
- Head
- Neck
- Body
- Tail

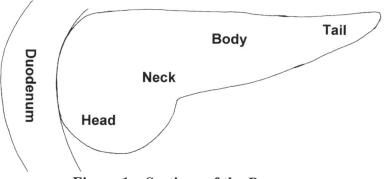

Figure 1—Sections of the Pancreas

2.3 Where's It Located?

In humans, the large head of the pancreas lies near the center of the abdomen—between the breastbone and the navel (bellybutton).

The head of the pancreas is attached to the first part of the small intestine (called the ***duodenum***). The back, or tapered tail end, of the pancreas lies next to the spleen and spine.

Figure 2 shows a diagram of the pancreas and its relationship to the duodenum (first part of the small intestine), liver, stomach, and gall bladder.

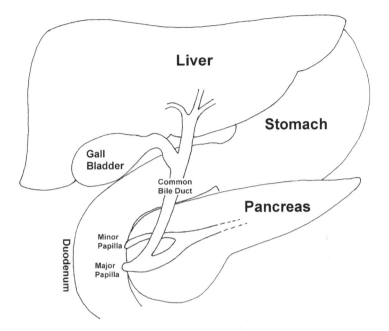

Figure 2—Major Digestive Organs of the Abdomen

In Figure 2, notice that the liver and gall bladder are connected to the pancreas via a branching, tree-like structure called the ***common bile duct*** (abbreviated CBD).

Now, let's briefly talk about ducts—you know, like the aluminum ducts that carry heat (and sometimes cool air) throughout your house, or maybe the building in which you work.

Your body has plenty of ducts, though they are made of live cells, not aluminum. The body's ducts come in many different sizes—some are large, some are small; some are called major, and so on.

The major ducts (discussed in more detail later) of the pancreas empty into the duodenum. These ducts are generally called pancreatic ducts (again, more on those later).

The two openings from the pancreatic ducts into the duodenum are called:

- the *minor papilla* (the top, smaller opening)
- the *major papilla* (the larger, bottom opening)

The pancreatic ducts and *papillae* (plural of papilla) drain the digestive juices (special chemicals called *enzymes*) from the pancreas into the small intestine to help digest food.

> By the way, the word papilla (pronounced *puh*-**PIL**-*uh*) is derived from the Latin word *papula*, which means nipple, teat, or pimple. In medical terms, a papilla is a nipple-like bulge, with a small hole in it.

Figure 3 shows a diagram of the *major papilla*. The major papilla is a bulge through the wall of the duodenum. The bulge is the end of one of the pancreatic ducts. There is a hole, surrounded by a circular muscle, in the papilla. This hole allows digestive enzymes to flow from the pancreas into the duodenum.

The hole and muscle around it are called the *Sphincter of Oddi*.

A *sphincter* is nothing more than a circular muscle surrounding a hole. When a sphincter contracts, it close the hole. When a sphincter relaxes, it opens the hole.

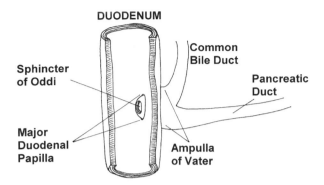

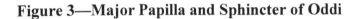

Figure 3—Major Papilla and Sphincter of Oddi

Origin:
The word sphincter (which is pronounced sfingk-**ter**) basically comes from the Greek word sphinktḗr, which means "something that holds tight."

This particular sphincter is named for the Italian physician Ruggero Oddi (prounced ŏd-dē), who discovered this sphincter muscle and hole while studying the action of bile on digestion.

2.4 What Does It Do?

The pancreas has two main functions—to produce and secrete...
- digestive chemicals (called *enzymes*) that break down fat, protein, and carbohydrates during digestion
- specialized chemicals (called *hormones*), such as glucagon and insulin, that aid-in the metabolism of sugars

2.4.1 Digestive Enzymes and Acinar Cells

The digestive enzymes are produced by specialized cells in the pancreas called the *acinar* (**as**-*in-ar*) cells. Groups or bunches of acinar cells form a small bundle called *acini* (**as**-*in-ee*). Figure 4 shows the acinar cells and acini.

The acinar cells secrete these digestive chemicals (enzymes) into the pancreatic ducts, which then empty into the duodenum.

The acinar cells are categorized as *exocrine* cells—cells that secrete chemicals directly into the ducts

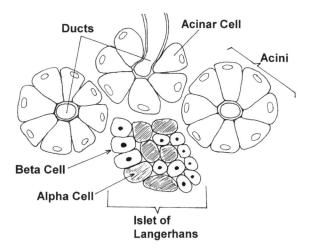

Figure 4—Pancreatic Endocrine and Exocrine Cells

Origin:
The word acinar is derived from the Latin word *acinus* (**as**-*in-us*), which means grape or berry.

2.4.2 Hormones and Islet Cells

The *hormones* (like insulin and glucagon) are produced by the *islet cells* of the pancreas. The hormones are released directly into the bloodstream. The islet cells are categorized as *endocrine* cells—meaning they secrete chemicals directly into the bloodstream.

A group or collection of islet cells is collectively known as the *Islet of Langerhans*.

> **Origin:**
> The Islet of Langerhans is named after the German anatomist Paul Langerhans who first discovered and described these cells.

Like acini, the islets are spread throughout the pancreas. Figure 4 also shows the islet cells and a collection of those cells in a bundle (the *Islet of Langerhans*).

The endocrine tissue—the Islets of Langerhans—consists of clusters of cells that manufacture the hormones insulin and glucagon. Insulin and glucagon work together to maintain the proper level of sugar (*glucose*) in your blood. Glucagon and insulin are secreted by the islet cells directly into the bloodstream.

Glucagon is used to raise very low blood sugar. Insulin allows cells in the liver, muscle, and fat tissue to take up glucose from the blood and store it for use as energy by the cells.

Destruction of the islets by your body's own immune system (white blood cells) results in type 1 (insulin-dependent) diabetes.

Failure of the islets to produce sufficient insulin or failure of your body's cells to absorb insulin from the bloodstream results in type 2 or non-insulin dependent (formerly called adult-onset) diabetes, or diabetes mellitus.

2.5 How's It Connected?

Ducts are tubes that transport chemicals and other substances from one part of the body to another. In the pancreas, the ducts transport digestive enzymes from the acinar cells to the duodenum.

The primary, and largest, duct is called the *main pancreatic duct* (shown in figure 5) The main pancreatic duct is a wide, long tube through the center of the pancreas that allows digestive enzymes from all parts of the pancreas to empty out into the small intestine to digest food.

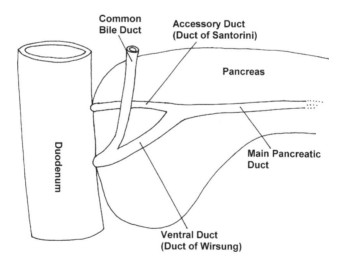

Figure 5—Major Ducts in the Pancreas

The pancreatic duct is also part of a tree-like structure called the *biliary system*. The biliary system (or tree) is comprised of a number of ducts and is shown in figure 6.

- *Hepatic Duct*: Originating in the liver, the hepatic duct transports *bile* to the gall bladder. Bile is a chemical, that helps digest fats. Until it is needed, the bile is stored in the gall bladder. The word hepatic is derived from the Greek word *hēpar*, which also means liver.
- *Cystic Duct*: The cystic duct allows bile to enter the gall bladder for storage. But, it also allows the gall bladder to send bile down into the digestive system for digestion. The bile is transported from the gall bladder through the cystic duct.
- *Common Bile Duct*: The cystic duct (from the gall bladder) and the hepatic duct (from the liver) merge to form the common bile duct (CBD). The common bile duct (CBD) then runs down to the pancreas where it joins with one of the pancreatic ducts. More on that later.

Figure 6 shows the cystic, hepatic, and common bile ducts.

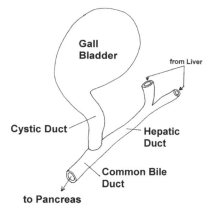

Labels on figure:
Gall Bladder
from Liver
Cystic Duct
Hepatic Duct
Common Bile Duct
to Pancreas

Figure 6—The Biliary Tree

2.6 Pancreatic Ductwork

Figure 7 shows the major ducts of the pancreas. Small, branch-like ducts from the acinar cells feed or connect into the major ducts of the pancreas.

The *main pancreatic duct* (MPD) splits into two smaller ducts, which then drain into the duodenum. These ducts are called the *accessory duct* (or, *duct of Santorini*) and the *ventral duct* (or, *duct of Wirsung*).

The tail and most of the body of the pancreas drain their digestive enzymes into the main pancreatic duct.

A small portion of the body and neck drain into the narrow accessory duct (the duct of Santorini). The rest of the neck and all of the head of the pancreas drain into the ventral pancreatic duct (duct of Wirsung).

Also, since the main pancreatic duct splits into the duct of Santorini and the duct of Wirsung, the enzymes (digestive juices) the MPD is carrying also drain into these ducts.

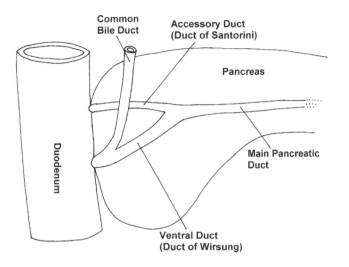

Figure 7—Ducts of the Pancreas

However, because the duct of Wirsung is much larger (wider) than the duct of Santorini, the majority of the enzymes from the MPD drain into the duct of Wirsung (the ventral pancreatic duct).

Origin:
The duct of Wirsung (pronounced *vir-sung*) is named after German anatomist Wirsung Johann Georg. Georg was a professor of anatomy in Padua, Italy. He discovered and drew an illustration of this particular duct.

The duct of Santorini is named for Italian anatomist Santorini Giovanni Domenico. He was a professor of anatomy and medicine in Venice, Italy. In a major work published in 1724, he described the accessory pancreatic duct. His works on anatomy provided thorough, detailed descriptions and precise graphic illustrations of human anatomy.

2.7 One Potential Problem

Now, as an aside (and, more on this later, I promise), herein lies the potential for a problem. There exists a *congenital* (at birth) defect known as *pancreas divisum*. This condition will be discussed in greater depth in a later section, but I just want to mention it briefly now.

In pancreas divisum, the ventral duct (Duct of Wirsung) does not merge or join with the accessory duct (Duct of Santorini) and the MPD (main pancreatic duct). In this case, the MPD drains solely into the narrow accessory duct (Santorini) while only the head of the pancreas drains into the much wider ventral duct (Wirsung).

Imagine what happens in this case.

> *A small amount of digestive juices easily drains out through the wide ventral duct. But, most of the fluids draining from the pancreas (tail, body, neck) are squeezed through the narrow accessory duct and out into the duodenum (first part of the small intestine). The pancreas has to work harder to squeeze these juices through the narrow accessory duct.*

It's like a never-ending traffic nightmare during rush hour! Think about this another way:

- The main pancreatic duct is a ten lane highway
- The accessory duct is a four lane highway
- The ventral duct is a ten lane highway
- All of these highways are one way (out of the pancreas)

In pancreas divisum, the 10-lane main pancreatic duct (MPD) narrows down to a 4-lane highway (the accessory duct)—what a traffic jam! While, on the other side of town, the 10-lane ventral duct is wide open—no traffic, no congestion.

Pancreatitis is inflammation or swelling of the pancreas. Damage to the pancreas can cause the pancreas to swell.

Swelling of the pancreas, in turn, can prevent digestive enzymes from secreting from the pancreas into the intestine.

The digestive enzymes, stuck inside the pancreas, then begin to digest the pancreas itself.

Notice, in figure 8, that the pancreas is so inflamed, its head is bulging into the duodenum, and the pancreatic ducts (main, ventral/Wirsung, and accessory/Santorini) are being squeezed shut due to the swelling of the pancreas.

The squeezing of the pancreatic ducts prevents digestive enzymes (from the acinar cells) from being able to drain from the pancreas. In turn, the enzymes, which are "activated" upon release from the acinar cells, build up in the pancreatic tissue and begin to digest the pancreas (known as ***autodigestion***). Instead of digesting food, the pancreas is digesting itself! Imagine the excruciating pain this can cause.

As the inflammation continues, and the acinar cells keep producing and activating digestive enzymes, the flood of digestive enzymes seeps around the islet cells and leaks into the bloodstream. Remember, the islet cells produce insulin and other hormones and release them directly into the bloodstream.

Once these activated digestive enzymes enter the bloodstream, they are carried all throughout the body. These digestive enzymes can settle anywhere.

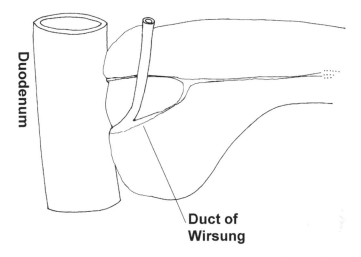

Duodenum

Duct of Wirsung

Figure 8—An Inflamed Pancreas and its Inflamed Ducts

Since they are active—ready to digest living tissue, such as food—they will digest anything. This is a big problem.

Imagine these digestive chemicals settling in your brain, heart, lungs, spine, kidneys, and other organs and tissues. Once there, the enzymes begin the process of digestion. Obviously, the result, over time, is destruction of these vital, life-sustaining organs.

It is this process that contributes significantly to the complications of pancreatitis and death to pancreatitis sufferers.

4. WHAT ARE THE TYPES OF PANCREATITIS?

There are two primary types or categories of pancreatitis:

- *acute pancreatitis*
- *chronic pancreatitis*

Other rarer forms include:

- *hereditary pancreatitis*
- *autoimmune pancreatitis*

The symptoms of these types of pancreatitis can mimic either acute or chronic pancreatitis, or both.

4.1 Acute Pancreatitis (AP)

4.1.1 What is AP?

Acute pancreatitis is a sudden attack of pain caused by inflammation of the pancreas. Sometimes, the tissue surrounding the pancreas can also become inflamed or swollen.

When the pancreas becomes inflamed, digestive enzymes cannot drain from the pancreas into the duodenum. Essentially, they become "stuck" in the pancreas.

Since these powerful chemicals—which help digest fats, proteins, and carbohydrates in the food passing through the small intestine—cannot get out of the pancreas, they begin to digest the pancreas itself. This leads to intense pain.

The enzymes can also "leak" into the bloodstream. The bloodstream then carries these digestive chemicals to other parts of the body where they can severely damage other organs such as the heart, lungs, and kidneys.

The sudden inflammation in acute pancreatitis can result in abdominal and back pain. The pain can range in intensity from mild discomfort to severe and crippling. The pain can last for a few minutes, a few hours, or a number of days.

Whereas a mild attack of acute pancreatitis usually results in abdominal pain and vomiting, a severe attack can result in...

- *Pancreatic necrosis*—death of pancreatic tissue
- *Systemic inflammation*—inflammation of organs and tissues throughout the body
- Shock
- Multiple organ failure

Acute pancreatitis is a very serious condition that can be life threatening. Each attack can lead to the damage or death of cells in the pancreas and other parts of your body.

However, prompt, proper medical treatment can usually relieve the symptoms and limit the damage from an attack.

In industrialized nations, the prevalence of acute pancreatitis is about 4 people per 100,000. (Löhr, 66). Fifty to eighty thousand cases of acute pancreatitis occur in the United States alone every year.

Table 1 lists the typical symptoms of acute pancreatitis.

Steady, boring upper abdominal pain	Patient appears acutely ill & sweaty
Pain in the back in 50% of patients	Pulse 100 - 140 beats per minutes
Temperature from normal to 101°F	BP fluctuates between high & low
Sitting up & leaning forward may decrease pain	Coughing, vigorous movement, or deep breathing increases pain
Pain that is sudden or develops over a few days; persists for several days	Person's senses are dulled to the point he/she seems to be in a semi-coma
Nausea & vomiting are common	Breathing is shallow & rapid
20% of patients have upper abdominal distension (swollen abdomen) due to gas or displacement of the stomach by pancreatic inflammation	

Table 1—Symptoms of AP

4.1.2 What Can Cause Acute Pancreatitis

The most common causes or triggers of acute pancreatitis are...

- Biliary tract disease—diseases of the gall bladder, common bile duct, or other parts of the organs and ducts involved with producing, storing, and secreting bile
- Chronic heavy alcohol intake

Biliary tract disease and alcoholism account for greater than 80% of acute pancreatitis cases.

Table 2 shows additional known or suspected triggers of acute pancreatitis.

Medications	Mechanical / Structural
ACE inhibitors	Gallstones
Asparaginase	ERCP
Azathioprine	Trauma
Pentamidine	Pancreatic cancer
Sulfa	Pancreas divisum
Valproate	Choledochal cyst
Furosemide	Narrowing (stenosis) or even obstructions of Sphincter of Oddi
Metabolic	**Infectious Agents**
Hypertriglyceridemia	Coxsackie B virus
Hypercalcemia	Cytomegalovirus
Hyperparathyroidism	Mumps
Estrogen Use	
Toxins	**Inherited (Genetic)**
Alcohol	Multiple known gene mutations
Methanol	Some of cystic fibrosis patients

Other
Pregnancy
Postrenal transplant
Tropical pancreatitis
Ischemia from hypotension
Ischemia from atheroembolism

Table 2—AP Triggers

Severe attacks of acute pancreatitis can lead to death (*necrosis*) of pancreatic cells and inflammation throughout the body. This, in turn, can lead to shock and failure of multiple organs including the kidneys (renal failure) and heart.

In acute pancreatitis, digestive enzymes become activated within the pancreas. These chemicals can damage cells and cause inflammation throughout the body. The inflammation can lead to swelling (*edema*).

In mild pancreatitis, the inflammation is confined to the pancreas. The *mortality* (death) rate is less than five percent.

In severe pancreatitis, there is a significant amount of inflammation. There can also be *necrosis* (death) of the pancreatic tissue, bleeding (*hemorrhaging*) of the pancreas itself, and body-wide (*systemic*) inflammation. Necrotic (dead) pancreatic tissue can become infected with bacteria. In severe pancreatitis, the mortality (death) rate can be as high as fifty percent.

The mortality rate for patients with an infected pancreas is about 100%, unless the pancreas is properly drained and antibiotics given. In some cases, surgical removal of dead and infected pancreatic tissue is necessary—this is called *debridement*.

About twenty percent of patients with severe pancreatitis become dehydrated and their blood pressure drops to dangerously low levels.

In about forty percent of patients, collections or pockets of pancreatic fluid and tissue debris (like dead cells) form in and around the pancreas. About fifty percent of these pockets resolve, or go away, spontaneously. In the remaining cases, these collections become infected or form *pseudocysts* (cyst-like pockets). The pseudocysts themselves are fibrous capsules that may bleed, rupture, or become infected.

Amylase is a digestive enzyme that breaks down starches. Lipase is a digestive enzymes that breaks down fat. In acute pancreatitis, the levels of amylase and lipase in the bloodstream are typically elevated, especially on the first day of the attack. Lipase and amylase levels return to normal three to seven days later.

However, if a sufficient number of acinar cells have been destroyed—and, therefore, cannot release sufficient amounts of enzymes—amylase and lipase levels in the blood may remain normal, since the pancreas will not be able to produce and secrete much of these enzymes.

Abdominal x-rays reveal *calcifications* (hardened areas of tissue) in the pancreatic ducts (which is evidence of chronic pancreatitis), calcified gallstones, and localized *ileus* (paralysis of part of the intestines).

An ultrasound can detect gallstones and dilation (widening) of the common bile duct (which indicates biliary tract obstruction).

A CT scan with contrast dye identifies necrosis, fluid collections, and pseudocysts.

4.2 Chronic Pancreatitis (CP)

Chronic pancreatitis is continued, ongoing (or very frequent) inflammation of the pancreas. In chronic pancreatitis, the swelling of the pancreas usually does not heal or improve and typically worsens over time. Chronic pancreatitis also typically leads to damage to the pancreas, which then becomes severely scarred. The damage cannot be reversed or repaired.

Chronic pancreatitis, which often develops in people between the ages of 30 and 40, typically occurs after one or more attacks of acute pancreatitis. Chronic pancreatitis can be brought on by a single acute attack that permanently damages the pancreas and pancreatic ducts.

In CP, scar tissue builds up in the pancreas, and the pancreas is slowly destroyed over time. Attacks of pain typically come and go in people afflicted with chronic pancreatitis. In many people with chronic pancreatitis, *calcification* (hardening) of the pancreas typically occurs within 8 to 10 years after the first symptoms appear.

In industrialized nations, the prevalence of chronic pancreatitis is 10 to 30 people per 100,000. As a side note, the prevalence of those with diabetes mellitus is 400 people per 100,000. (Löhr, 66)

70% of chronic pancreatitis cases are due to alcohol abuse—people averaging three to four drinks per day over ten years. The life expectancy of people with advanced pancreatitis is typically shortened by ten to twenty years. The link between alcohol abuse and pancreatitis was first noticed in 1878 by Nikolaus Friedreich, a German physician, pathologist, and neurologist.

4.3 Hereditary Pancreatitis

Less common than the other two types is *hereditary pancreatitis*. This condition is a rare, inherited (i.e., genetic) condition that is usually passed from one generation to the next in families.

Hereditary pancreatitis is likely if you have two or more family members with pancreatitis in more than one generation. It is characterized by recurring attacks of acute pancreatitis. About 50% of people with hereditary pancreatitis develop chronic pancreatitis as a result of the recurring attacks. In the U.S., at least 1,000 people are affected with hereditary pancreatitis.

4.4 Autoimmune Pancreatitis

Another (although very rare) form of pancreatitis is *autoimmune pancreatitis*—a term first used in Japan in 1995. It is a form of chronic pancreatitis. The symptoms can closely resemble those of pancreatic cancer. This makes diagnosing autoimmune pancreatitis difficult.

There are a few methods for detecting autoimmune pancreatitis:

- Imaging—such as CT scan or MRI
- Endoscopic pancreatic core biopsy—a non-surgical method of obtaining a sample of pancreatic tissue using an endoscope; doctors then look at the tissue under a microscope; autoimmune pancreatitis has a distinctive appearance
- Blood test to detect IgG4—this is a protein (actually, an antibody) in your blood; elevated levels can indicate autoimmune pancreatitis

Autoimmune pancreatitis can affect not only the pancreas but also the lymph nodes, kidneys, and bile ducts. It occurs when your body's own immune system mistakenly attacks healthy organs. This causes inflammation and eventual destruction of the cells.

Corticosteroids (such as prednisone) can reduce the inflammation and damage to the cells. However, frequent relapses can still occur.

5. WHAT ARE THE SYMPTOMS OF PANCREATITIS?

5.1 The Symptoms

The most common, and almost always present, symptom of pancreatitis is abdominal pain. This pain usually occurs in the upper center of the abdomen (like a sharp stabbing pain in the stomach).

The pain can be aggravated by eating (especially fatty foods) or drinking anything—even water. Walking or lying down can also aggravate the pain, while leaning or bending forward frequently relieves the pain. Your abdomen can become swollen and tender. Many people also experience sharp back pain in the center or just to the left of the center of the back.

The pain can be constant and disabling.

In chronic pancreatitis sufferers, the pain may eventually disappear altogether once the pancreas becomes so damaged that it stops producing digestive enzymes.

Table 3 provides an extensive but not exhaustive list of other symptoms of pancreatitis. Not everyone will experience all of these symptoms.

Abdominal tenderness & rigidity	Hypotension (low blood pressure)
Bluish discoloration of the abdomen due to bleeding from the pancreas	Jaundice (yellow eyes/skin)
Weight loss due to poor digestion and malnutrition	Muscle spasms in arms and legs (low calcium level)
Chills	Nausea and/or Vomiting
Clammy (cold, sweaty skin)	Rapid pulse or heart rate
Dehydration	Sweating
Diarrhea	Tiredness
Diminished or absent bowel sounds	Fever
Dyspepsia	Weakness
Fatty or oily stools	Bloating

Table 3—Symptoms of Pancreatitis

5.2 Immediate Medical Concerns

There are a number of immediate medical concerns in pancreatitis.

If you have any of the symptoms of pancreatitis, especially sharp, stabbing abdominal pain, you should see a doctor or go to a hospital emergency room immediately.

A person with acute pancreatitis usually looks and feels very ill and needs immediate medical attention.

Severe acute pancreatitis can cause heart, lung, and kidney failure, and bleeding in the pancreas can lead to shock and death.

Fat necrosis—death of fat cells around the pancreas—can cause *hypocalcemia,* which is a low calcium level in the blood. A drop in calcium can cause the heart to function poorly.

Also, damage to the islets or beta cells can cause hyperglycemia (high blood sugar) and lead to diabetes.

6. WHAT ARE THE CAUSES OF PANCREATITIS?

There are a number of different causes of pancreatitis:

- alcoholism
- infection
- heredity (genetics)
- certain drugs/medications

In many cases, there is no identifiable cause at all—this is called *idiopathic*.

6.1 Alcoholism

The most common cause of chronic pancreatitis is alcoholism.

In more than 70% of cases, chronic pancreatitis is caused by long-term alcohol use. Many years of heavy alcohol use scars and damages the pancreas.

The exact effects of alcohol on the pancreas are neither well known nor understood. However, byproducts of ethanol (drinking alcohol) can damage the acinar cells—and this can lead to inflammation of the pancreas.

6.2 Gallstones

The most common cause of acute pancreatitis is *gallstones*—small, pebble-like substances made of hardened bile or cholesterol.

The inflammation is usually caused by one of two gallstone happenings:

- a gallstone that is passing through the common bile duct (see figure 9) irritates and inflames the pancreas
- a gallstone becomes stuck in the biliary tract and blocks the exit of enzymes from the pancreas, thereby causing the pancreas to swell

Figure 9 shows how the common bile duct is formed by the merger of the cystic duct (from the gall bladder) and the hepatic duct (from the liver). The common bile duct then merges with the ventral pancreatic duct (duct of Wirsung).

Gallstones can get stuck at any point along this path. Gallstones can get stuck in the neck of the gall bladder, in the cystic duct, or in the common bile duct and cause acute attacks of pain (gall bladder attacks or *cholecystitis*).

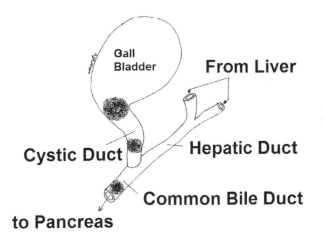

Figure 9—Gall Stones in the Biliary Tree

n also become stuck at the junction of the
reatic duct and the common bile duct, and this
pancreatitis. See figure 10.

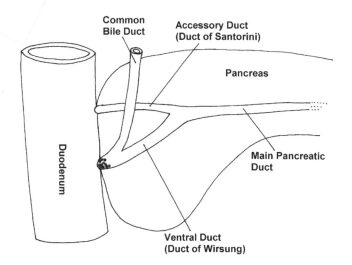

**Figure 10—Gall Stones Blocking the Ventral Pancreatic
Duct**

6.3 Infections

A number of different infections can cause pancreatitis.
These include the viruses that cause *mumps* and *coxsackie
B* as well as the *campylobacter* and *mycoplasma
pneumonia* bacteria.

6.4 Medications

Many medications are *suspected* of causing pancreatitis in
some people. Some medications may not cause pancreatitis
but can potentially worsen the disease. Table 5 lists
medications that have been reported to cause or are
suspected of causing or worsening pancreatitis.

Advair	Estrogens
Azathioprine	Statins (e.g., Lipitor)
Byetta	Januvia (Sitagliptin)
Corticosteroids (such as prednisone)	Thiazide diuretics (e.g., HCTZ)
Depakote (Valproate)	Xenical

Table 5—Medications That May Cause/Worsen Pancreatitis

6.5 Pancreas Divisum

Pancreas divisum is a congenital defect in the structure of the pancreas. This means that a person with pancreas divisum is born with this condition (that is, it's ***congenital***).

Pancreas divisum means that the two major pieces of the pancreas (the ventral section and the dorsal section) do not merge or fuse to form a single, contiguous pancreas gland. In other words, the pancreas remains "divided" into two sections (hence the term divisum).

Pancreas divisum affects about 7 to 10% of the population. "Autopsy studies estimate the prevalence of PD at 5-10%."

Here's how this anomaly occurs.

In the early stages of development of the ***fetus*** (the yet-unborn "baby"), the pancreas exists as two separate structures (see figure 11). These separate pieces are known as the ventral bud (or, ***anlage***) and the dorsal bud (or, anlage). An ***anlage*** (pronounced **ahn**-lah-*guh*) is an organ in its earliest stage of development as a cluster of cells.

These two pieces of pancreatic tissue form on opposite sides of what will become the ***duodenum*** (first part of the small intestine). Again, see figure 11.

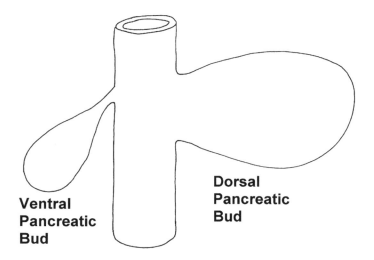

Ventral
Pancreatic
Bud

Dorsal
Pancreatic
Bud

Figure 11—Early Stage of Pancreas Development:
Separate Ventral and Dorsal Buds

As the fetus grows, the ventral pancreatic bud moves toward the dorsal pancreatic bud (shown in figures 12 and 13), that is, it rotates clockwise around the duodenum.

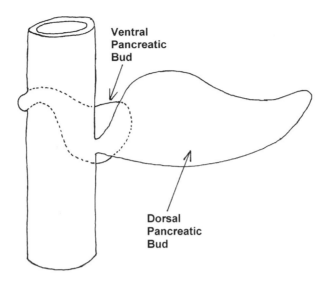

Ventral
Pancreatic
Bud

Dorsal
Pancreatic
Bud

**Figure 12—Early Stage of Pancreas Development:
Rotating Ventral Bud**

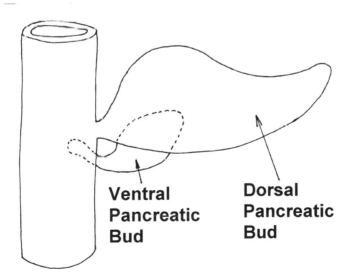

**Ventral
Pancreatic
Bud**

**Dorsal
Pancreatic
Bud**

**Figure 13—Early Stage of Pancreas Development:
Ventral Bud Begins Fusion with Dorsal Bud**

As the fetus continues to grow, sometime during or around the eighth week of development, the ventral and dorsal buds (or, anlage) merge to form a single gland—the pancreas. During the fusion process, the ventral and dorsal ducts join—see figure 14.

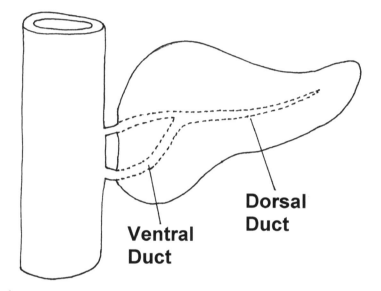

**Figure 14—Early Stage of Pancreas Development:
Fusion of Ventral and Dorsal Buds Completed**

However, sometimes the process just stops (for reasons unknown) before the fusion has completed. The baby is then born with a pancreas that has not properly fused. As a result, the two ducts (one from each part of the original two structures) never join. This is pancreas divisum, which is shown in figure 15.

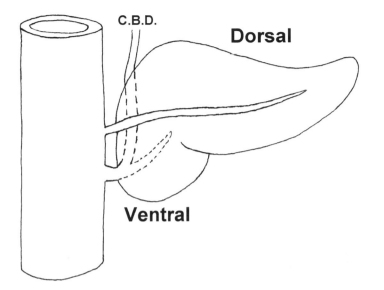

Figure 15—Pancreas Divisum: Incomplete Fusion of the Ventral and Dorsal Buds

Figure 16 shows, as we have seen before, a properly fused and formed pancreas.

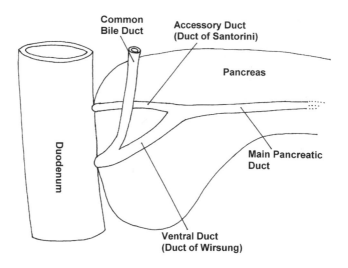

Figure 16—Pancreatic Ducts and Common Bile Duct

Now, a little more anatomy on the structure of the pancreas, so you can understand why pancreas divisum could be or become a problem.

First of all, a properly constructed, fused pancreas results in the following structures:

- The first part of the dorsal duct is known as the accessory duct or duct of Santorini
- The latter part of the dorsal duct is known as the main pancreatic duct
- The ventral duct (or, duct of Wirsung) connects the main pancreatic duct to the duodenum
- The duct of Santorini drains into the duodenum through a small hole called the minor papilla
- The duct of Wirsung drains into the duodenum through a large hold called the major papilla

- The common bile duct joins with the duct of Wirsung—this juncture point is called the ampulla of Vater (see figure 17)

The main pancreatic duct and the duct of Wirsung:
- Is a wide duct
- Starts at the tip of the tail
- Ends at the major duodenal papilla in the duodenum
- Drains exocrine secretions from the head, body, and tail of the pancreas
- Also joins with the common bile duct to form the ampulla of Vater (see figure 17)

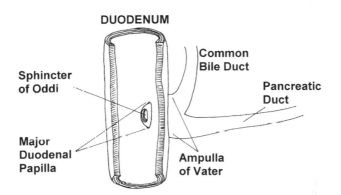

Figure 17—Pancreatic Ducts and Common Bile Duct

The accessory pancreatic duct or duct of Santorini:
- Is a narrow duct
- Is used for overflow of enzymes
- Extends through the head of the pancreas
- Crosses the duct of Wirsung
- Ends at the minor duodenal papilla

In a properly constructed pancreas, where the ventral and dorsal ducts have joined, most of the pancreatic juices drain via the larger ventral duct (duct of Wirsung).

The accessory duct (the duct of Santorini) is narrow and serves only to drain some excess or overflow juices through the minor papilla.

Now, here's the problem with pancreas divisum. Because the narrow duct of Santorini is in the larger part of the pancreas, it's draining the majority of pancreatic juices from the pancreas into the duodenum. This duct is short and narrow and therefore was not designed or built to handle this much flow.

This part of the pancreas eventually becomes damaged by the juices not getting out of the pancreas fast enough. The build-up of juices also causes damage to the pancreas itself and the pancreas becomes swollen and inflamed.

The wide duct of Wirsung has no problem draining, but because it never connected to the rest of the pancreas, it's only draining the small head of the pancreas, and there's not much flowing out of that area.

So in pancreas divisum, the ventral duct (Wirsung) is a wide-open ten-lane highway with little or no traffic, while the accessory duct (Santorini) is a narrow, dirt back road that allows only one car to pass through at a time!

Years and years of this backwards functioning eventually, in many people, damages the pancreas beyond repair. The result can be damage to the acinar cells, damage to the islet cells, acute attacks of pancreatitis, chronic pancreatitis, extreme pain, and eventual death of the organ due to auto or self digestion.

The auto or self-digestion is caused when the activated digestive enzymes get stuck in the pancreas (instead of flowing into the intestines) and start to digest the pancreas itself! Worse yet, these powerful digestive enzymes can leak into the bloodstream where they are carried to other parts of the body. Then, the enzymes (looking for tissue to digest) can eat away at the brain, heart, lungs, kidneys, liver, and so on. Imagine the damage (and pain) that causes!

There are actually three types of pancreas divisum:

1. Classic scenario: there is no connection between the ventral and dorsal ducts
2. Incomplete fusion: there is a very narrow duct joining the ventral and dorsal ducts
3. The duct of Wirsung may be completely absent

Not all people with pancreas divisum (PD) will show symptoms of or suffer from pancreatitis. "Although the prevalence of PD in the general population is relatively high, only a small proportion of those with congenital anomaly will develop symptoms of pancreas divisum during their lifetime."

Diet and pancreatic enzymes can help people who experience symptoms of pancrcatitis due to pancreas divisum. A minor surgical procedure, known as a *sphincterotomy*, can also help. In a sphincterotomy, a physician makes a cut in the minor papilla to allow the duct of Wirsung to drain. Typically, a stent (like a short tube) is placed in the cut to hold the hole open long enough for the duct to drain.

The stent eventually (usually in less than a week) falls out, into the intestines, and is passed out of the body. If the stent remains in place, it too can become clogged and cause further attacks of pancreatitis. (In this case, the physician would need to remove the stent). The sphincterotomy is performed using an **endoscope**—a thin, lighted tube passed down the throat, through the stomach, and into the duodenum.

6.6 Annular Pancreas

Annular pancreas is a rare, **congenital** (born with it) anomaly. It occurs when the ventral pancreatic bud wraps itself around the duodenum (small intestine) instead of merging with the dorsal pancreatic bud during growth of the fetus.

About 1 in 2000 people has annular pancreas. Annular pancreas can occur either by itself or with other congenital anomalies. People with annular pancreas can have symptoms of pancreatitis, peptic ulcer disease, or duodenal obstruction. Annular pancreas is diagnosed using MRI or CT scan.

There are two types of annular pancreas:

a) *Extramural*—where the ventral pancreatic duct encircles the duodenum and joins the main pancreatic duct

b) *Intramural*—where pancreatic tissue intermingles with muscle fibers in the small intestine and small ducts drain directly into the duodenum.

6.7 Other Causes of Pancreatitis

Other known or suspected causes of pancreatitis include…

- Smoking
- Surgery of or around the pancreas or common bile duct
- Traumatic injury to the pancreas (such as injury to the abdomen in an automobile accident)
- The gene mutation responsible for cystic fibrosis increases the risk of pancreatitis (both acute and chronic)

6.8 Idiopathic Pancreatitis

In some cases, the cause of pancreatitis is not known or cannot be identified. This is known as *idiopathic pancreatitis*. It occurs in about 10 to 15% of pancreatitis sufferers.

7. How is Pancreatitis Diagnosed?

There are a number of different tests and procedures used to identify and diagnose pancreatitis. In addition to these tests, genetic testing can help doctors identify hereditary pancreatitis.

7.1 Blood Test (Lab Tests or Laboratory Studies)

Perhaps the easiest and most common diagnostic tests used to identify suspected pancreatitis are blood tests. When blood is drawn and sent to the lab for analysis, doctors usually look for the following indicators of pancreas problems:

Amylase
- A sugar-digesting enzyme manufactured in the pancreas
- Is usually 3 or more times higher than normal
- Normal Range: 23 to 85 units per liter

Blood glucose
- Measures how much sugar is circulating in the blood
- Indicates B or islet cell damage
- Normal Range: < 100 milligrams per deciliter

Blood Urea Nitrogen (BUN)
- Elevated
- BUN test measures the amount of nitrogen in the blood that comes from the waste product urea (produced during the breakdown of proteins)
- Normal Range: 7 to 20 milligrams per deciliter

CA-19 or CA 19-9
- An indicator of possible pancreatic cancer
- Normal range: 0 to 37 units per milliliter

C-Reactive Protein (CRP)
- Produced by the liver
- Elevated when there is inflammation throughout the body
- Normal Range: generally, no detectable level in the blood

Creatinine
- Elevated level indicates kidney damage
- Normal Range: 0.8 to 1.4 milligrams per deciliter

Electrolytes
- Sodium, potassium, chlorine, carbon dioxide, phosphorus, magnesium
- Usually a great imbalance among these

Glucose Tolerance Test
- Another blood sugar test that measures damage to the islet cells

Immunoglobulin G4 (IgG4)
- An indicator of inflammation

Lipase
- A fat-digesting enzyme manufactured in the pancreas
- Elevated and may remain high for up to 12 days
- Normal Range: 0 to 160 units per liter

Trypsin
- Most accurate indicator of acute pancreatitis
- Not available in many labs
- A pancreatic enzyme used to help break down proteins
- Normal range: < 100 micrograms per Liter

White Blood Count (WBC)
- May be > 12000 if infection is present
- Normal range: 4500-10000 white blood cells per microliter

7.2 Radiographic Studies

In addition to blood tests, a number of radiographic (x-ray like) procedures can be used to diagnose pancreatitis.

7.2.1 X-Rays

- Abdomen and chest
- Typically performed to rule out any other problems first (such as large gas bubbles in the intestine or an enlarged heart)

7.2.2 Contrast-Enhanced Computerized Tomography (CT) Scan

- Type of X-ray device that uses a donut-shaped machine to produce three-dimensional pictures of the inside of the body
- Provides best images of pancreas and surrounding structures
- Used to rule out causes of acute and chronic pancreatitis (such as gallstones and pseudocysts)
- Does not reliably detect pancreas divisum

7.2.3 Abdominal Ultrasound

- A hand-held device (sort of like a microphone) that sends sound waves through the abdomen
- Sound waves bounce off the pancreas, gall bladder, and liver and are transferred to a video monitor that creates a picture (called a *sonogram*) of these organs
- Would typically show gallstones

7.2.3 Endoscopic Ultrasound (EUS)

- Uses an endoscope (a thin, flexible, lighted tube) inserted down the throat, through the stomach, and into the small intestine
- Ultrasound device is attached to the scope to generate sound waves to create a picture of the pancreas and bile ducts

7.2.6 Secretin-Stimulated Diffusion-Weight MRI

- Recently developed non-invasive procedure
- Used to evaluate functioning of the acinar cells
- May also help to detect mild pancreatitis via changes in the structure of the pancreas and its smaller side ducts.

7.2.4 Endoscopic Retrograde Cholangiopancreatography (ERCP)

- Uses X-rays, an endoscope, and contrast dye to look at the pancreas, pancreatic ducts, and bile ducts
- Shows gallstones as well as deformities of and damage to the pancreas
- Is the "gold standard" for detecting chronic pancreatitis (even mild CP)
- Allows physician to see changes in pancreatic ducts, even when subtle
- Is invasive—therefore, it has a high risk for complications (such as causing acute pancreatitis)
- Is a difficult procedure to perform and requires a very experienced physician
- Cannot be used to assess functioning of the acini
- Can be used to see pancreas divisum

- During ERCP treatment, options for patients with pancreas divisum include:
  - Sphincterotomy of minor papilla—cutting the sphincter muscle
  - Papillary dilatation—dilating or expanding the minor papilla opening
  - Inserting a stent into the minor papilla opening

- Other procedures during ERCP:
  - Stone extraction—removal of pancreatic duct stones
  - Extracorporeal shockwave lithotripsy (ESWL) with stone extraction—that is, using powerful radio waves to shatter the stones and then pick up the pieces
  - Dilation (widening) of the beginning part of the pancreatic duct

- Possible complications during ERCP:
  - Pain after the procedure
  - Pancreatitis attacks after the procedure

- Post-ERCP Pancreatitis
  - Increased amylase level is common after ERCP in up to 75% of patients
  - Most serious complication is attack of (acute) pancreatitis
  - Severe & even fatal pancreatitis can occur after diagnostic ERCP
  - Incidence of post-ERCP pancreatitis is 1.6% to 17.7% (Munoz & Katerdahl)
- Causes of post-ERCP pancreatitis include injury to the pancreatic duct from:
  - Instrumentation
  - Prolonged manipulation around papillary opening

- o Multiple injections of dye into the pancreatic duct
- o Allergy to the contrast dye
- o Irritation from the contrast dye
- o Injury from enzymes backing up into the pancreas from the duodenum
- o Infection & bacterial injury from contaminated endoscope & accessories

7.2.5 Magnetic Resonance Cholangiopancreatography (MRCP)

- Limited availability and high cost
- Rapidly becoming the non-invasive test of choice to diagnose pancreas divisum
- Uses an MRI machine and contrast dye (injected into a vein) to show problems in the pancreas, gall bladder, bile ducts, and pancreatic ducts, much like the ERCP
- It's non-invasive—it is safe with no adverse effects
- Usually clearly shows problems with the major pancreatic duct (such as dilatation and stricture)
- Allows visualization of stones, protein plugs, pseudocysts, and the pancreatic ducts
- Involves no radiation
- Is an easy procedure to perform
- Does not show mild changes in the smaller pancreatic branch ducts
- Can show pancreas divisum and annular pancreas
- Used to diagnose moderate to severe pancreatitis (however, usually cannot be used to diagnose mild pancreatitis)

8. WHAT ARE THE COMPLICATIONS OF PANCREATITIS?

8.1 Overview of Complications

Because of the effects of chronic pancreatitis, the damaged pancreas becomes less able over time to produce normal digestive enzymes and hormones. The constant inflammation or swelling of the pancreas and the resulting damage can lead to complications. Table 6 lists some of the more common complications experienced by chronic pancreatitis sufferers.

Abscesses, cysts, & infections	Damage to other organs
Bleeding	Inability to digest food
Chronic pain	Diabetes
Scarring of the pancreas	

Table 6—Potential Complications of Chronic Pancreatitis

One of the most dangerous complications of chronic pancreatitis is the destruction of other organs in the body.

Recall the basic discussion about the pancreas' anatomy. The acinar cells (which produce digestive enzymes) drain into the pancreatic ducts, which then drain into the duodenum (first part of the small intestine).

The alpha and beta cells (which produce hormones including insulin) drain directly into the bloodstream. When the pancreas becomes inflamed and the digestive enzymes are unable to drain from the pancreatic duct into the small intestine, the enzymes build up and then back up into the pancreas.

The digestive enzymes then overrun the alpha cells (which will digest and destroy those cells over time and lead to diabetes). As the alpha and beta cells are flooded, the runoff drains into the bloodstream.

These potent and powerful digestive enzymes are then carried by the bloodstream to other parts of the body where they can digest and destroy the heart, lungs, kidneys, and other vital organs. This can lead to acute renal (kidney) failure, heart failure, shock, and death.

- About 20 to 30% of patients with acute pancreatitis (AP) develop complications of necrosis, organ failure, or both
- Most complications of AP, and subsequent deaths, occur within 2 weeks of pain onset
- 70 to 80% of deaths from pancreatitis are due to secondary pancreas infection (the most common cause of death in AP)
- Complications include necrosis and organ failure (cardiovascular, pulmonary, renal)
- Pseudocysts occur in 1 to 8% of cases
- Abscesses occur in 1 to 4% of cases
- Diabetes mellitus is a common result (from destruction of the islet cells by digestive enzymes)
- Jaundice (which is an indicator that the liver has been severely damaged)

8.2 Fibrosing Colonopathy

Fibrosing colonopathy is severe thickening of the wall of the large intestine (colon). It causes abdominal pain, distension (swollen abdomen), vomiting, and constipation.

Fibrosing colonopathy has recently been described as a complication in pancreatitis patients who have cystic fibrosis. (CF)

Fibrosing colonopathy typically appears in CF patients about 7 to 12 months after they start high doses of pancreatic enzymes (supplements). Research studies have indicated that there is a high correlation between fibrosing colonopathy and the dose of pancreatic enzyme.

There are a number of suspected reasons why pancreatic enzymes can cause fibrosing colonopathy:

a) Certain specific pancreatic enzymes may be toxic and cause damage to the cells of the colon
b) The substance which coats the capsule or tablet of pancreatic enzymes may be damaging to the colon
c) There may be impurities in the pancreatic enzyme extracts which damage the colon
d) Ingestion of high concentrations of pancreatic enzymes could be setting off an immune response (like an allergic reaction)

8.3 Pancreatic Psudeocysts

A cyst is a closed sac of cells with a distinct wall (membrane). Cysts usually contain fluid, air, or semi-solid material.

A pseudocyst is a collection of fluid inside a sac made of Jello-like material or fibrous tissue (not a true membrane like around a cyst). Pseudocysts often appear to be actual cysts, even on a CT scan. Laboratory studies are used to determine whether or not a cystic-like object is a cyst or pseudocyst.

Pseudocysts are the most common type of cysts in the pancreas. They can be surgically drained or they may just go away on their own. They typically develop as a complication of alcoholic, biliary, or traumatic acute pancreatitis.

Blood tests consistently show higher levels of amylase when pseudocysts are present.

8.4 Malnutrition

Malnutrition can occur when the acinar cells become too damaged to produce any more digestive enzymes.

Then, protein and fat pass through the small intestine largely undigested. These globs of partially digested fat and protein then pass into the large intestine (colon).

Eventually, the globs of undigested fat irritate the walls of the colon and can lead to problems such as steatorrhea, malnutrition, and irritable bowel. Steatorrhea is greasy, oily *poop*.

Malnutrition is seen in about 30% of people with chronic pancreatitis. Malnutrition can contribute significantly to weight loss and muscle wasting. Malnutrition can also prevent the body from properly repairing wounds (cuts, scrapes, and so on) because the proteins and nutrients needed for repair are not available to the skin.

8.5 Hypotension

Hypotension is abnormally low blood pressure.

When the body's blood flow is too low, sufficient blood does not get to the heart, brain, and other vital organs.

Lack of blood flow from hypotension can cause dizziness and lightheadedness.

Severe inflammation of organs (such as the pancreas) can cause low blood pressure. In acute pancreatitis, for example, fluid leaves the blood to enter the inflamed tissues around the pancreas and throughout the abdomen. This causes depletion or reduction of blood in the rest of the body and, in turn, causes the blood pressure to drop.

9. HOW IS PANCREATITIS TREATED?

9.1 Overview of Treatments

Treatment for an attack of pancreatitis can range from basic to intensive, depending upon…

- the severity of the attack
- the amount of damage to the pancreas
- the amount of pain the patient experiences

Treatment typically includes at least some of the following…

- Antibiotics—which can improve the outcome of patients with severe disease and can prevent infections in pancreatic necrosis
- Fluids—IV fluids with electrolytes, since inadequate fluids increases the risk of pancreatic necrosis (death of pancreas cells)
- Fasting— a few days to several weeks
- TPN to prevent malnutrition if pancreatitis is severe
- Pain relief—usually narcotic pain killers; however, morphine may cause Sphincter of Oddi contractions and spasms, thus increasing pain
- Antiemetics—to alleviate vomiting
- Naso-gastric tube (NGT)—for persistent vomiting or ileus (paralytic ileus—when part of the bowel/large intestine just stops working)
- Medications to decrease stomach acid
- Humidified oxygen (if oxygen levels are low)
- Drainage of pseudocysts
- Surgical debridement of pseudocysts—that is, surgically removing dead, damaged, or infected

tissue to help the remaining healthy tissue to heal or prevent it from becoming damaged
- ERCP with sphincterotomy for stone removal
- Special diet (usually low-fat and low-calorie) with pancreatic enzyme supplements

9.2 Treating with Fluids

First and foremost in treating any type of pancreatitis are…

- Fluid resuscitation (putting water back into your body)
- Pain control

A person suffering from an attack of acute pancreatitis is unable to eat or drink anything, because anything put into the mouth would worsen the attack by "stimulating" the pancreas. Therefore, water must be given intravenously (by IV). Dehydration (lack of water) worsens pancreatitis and can lead to shock and death.

Pain control (using narcotics such as hydromorphone or meperidine) provides comfort to the pain by alleviating the pain of the attack. Pain is the most debilitating symptom in 90% of patients with chronic pancreatitis.

9.3 Treating for Fluid Build-up and Infections

If signs of infection are present—such as an elevated white blood cell count—antibiotics would typically be administered to destroy the bacteria causing the infection.

Otherwise, the bacteria could spill from the pancreas into the bloodstream and cause septic shock. Septic shock is a serious medical condition caused by severe low blood pressure and decreased oxygen in the tissues and organs as a result of widespread infection throughout the body. Septic shock can lead to multiple organ failure (and, obviously, death).

If parts of the pancreas are severely damaged or pancreatic tissue has died, fluid could build up in the organ. This fluid causes pressure, which results in an increase in pain. The fluid could also harbor bacteria, which could lead to infection and septic shock. In this case, a CT scan and needle are used to drain the fluid from the pancreas.

9.4 Treating for Gallstones

If pancreatitis is due to gallstones, an ERCP procedure can be used to remove the stones.

9.5 Treating Pain

For patients experiencing unrelenting pain in chronic pancreatitis, one option is a *pancreatectomy*—total removal of the pancreas

This option has two primary benefits…

- It stops the pain being caused by the damaged pancreas
- It prevents further damage to organs outside the pancreas

The dramatic disadvantage…

- The patient will no longer have a pancreas to produce insulin and digestive enzymes
- The patient would require insulin injections, blood sugar monitoring, and pancreatic enzyme supplements for the rest of his or her life.

option is surgical resection of the removal of parts of the pancreas

A third option is ongoing treatment with powerful narcotic painkillers. The disadvantages include …

- Addiction
- Necessity of constant use
- Side effects of narcotics
- Loss of effectiveness over time
- Doesn't prevent pancreatic damage from worsening

On a more positive note, greater than 80% of people with acute pancreatitis recover completely with the correct treatments.

9.6 Treatment Via Diet

Aside from blood tests and medical procedures, diet also plays a major part in controlling pancreatitis.

9.6.1 Low Fat Diet

A low-fat diet may be helpful to those with pancreatitis, since damage to the pancreas reduces its ability to secrete fat-digesting enzymes.

In addition, a diet comprised mainly of soft foods and liquids may be beneficial, as these types of foods require less pancreatic enzymes for digestion.

9.6.2 Calorie-Restricted Diet

Recent scientific studies have also found that a low-calorie or calorie-restricted diet reduces pancreatic inflammation.

A reduction in pancreatic inflammation greatly decreases scarring of the pancreas (which also decreases the possibility of pancreatic cancer).

In addition, fat stored in the body releases chemicals called *cytokines*, which cause inflammation throughout the body and contribute to additional pain. Therefore, a reduction of fat reduces cytokines that, in turn, reduces inflammation.

Try to remember this:

$\downarrow$ **calories** $\Rightarrow$ $\downarrow$ **fat** $\Rightarrow$ $\downarrow$ **cytokines** $\Rightarrow$ $\downarrow$ **inflammation** $\Rightarrow$ $\downarrow$ **pain**

People with pancreatitis should also eat small, frequent meals to reduce the strain on the pancreas. They should also keep well hydrated by drinking plenty of water.

Pancreatitis sufferers should not smoke or drink any alcoholic beverages, regardless of the extent or severity of the pancreatitis. Both smoking and alcohol can significantly worsen pancreatitis.

9.6.3 Pancreatic Enzymes

For people whose digestive ability is compromised by pancreatitis, pancreatic enzymes are usually necessary. Pancreatic enzymes are pills or capsules that contain the chemicals needed to digest fats, carbohydrates, and protein.

These products contain *pancrealipase*—a pancreatic enzyme mix of lipase, protease, and amylase (all derived from pigs):

- Lipase—used for digesting fats
- Protease--used for digesting proteins
- Amylase—used for digesting carbohydrates

Although pancreatic enzyme supplements are required for those with severely damaged pancreases, there can be unpleasant and sometimes serious side effects from pancrealipase. Table 7 lists some of these side effects.

Anaphylaxis *	Dizziness
Abdominal pain	High uric acid ("gout")
Constipation	Nausea
Coughing	Rashes
Diarrhea	Weight Loss

Table 7—Side Effects of Pancrealipase

Anaphylaxis is probably the most serious side effect of taking pancrealipase. Anaphylaxis is a rapid-onset, severe allergic reaction that can induce asthma attacks, cause swelling of body parts (eyes, mouth, throat), and cause hives and pruritus (non-stop itching).

If you experience any of these side effects, or any of the side effects listed in Table 8, go to a hospital emergency room or call 9-1-1 (or the emergency number in your area) immediately. These side effects are signs of a severe allergic reaction to the pancreatic enzymes and can be life-threatening.

Anxiety; feeling of doom	Itchy mouth/throat/eyes
Chest pain / tightness	Lightheadedness
Diarrhea	Low or slow pulse
Dizziness	Nausea
Drop in blood pressure	Pale or blue skin color (low oxygen)
Flushing (turning bright or beet red)	Severe abdominal pains / cramps
Fainting	Shortness of breath
Headache	Stuffy or congested nose
Heart attack	Swelling face/tongue/throat
Hives	Throat tightness
Hoarse Voice	Trouble swallowing
Irregular heartbeat	Vomiting
Itching	Wheezing

Table 8—*Signs of Anaphylaxis (quick, severe allergic reaction)

Like other allergies, reactions to the medication can be severe. If you have several of the symptoms listed in Table 8 or if your symptoms are severe, you should seek immediate medical attention in a hospital.

9.7 Treating for Pancreas Divisum

9.7.1 Treating the Symptoms Caused by Pancreas Divisum

- Pain relief (known as parenteral analgesia, or pain medications via I.V.)
- No food or liquids by mouth for at least a few days
- No alcohol (at all)
- Diet changes (low fat; reduced calorie, as mentioned before)
- Pancreatic enzyme supplements (as mentioned before)
- Hydration with fluids, that is, keep hydrated with lots of water (parenterally—via I.V.—at first, then eventually by mouth)
- Minor papilla sphincterotomy (see details below)

9.7.2 Minor Papilla Sphincterotomy [MPS]

- MPS is the making of a small cut in the minor papilla to widen the sphincter (the hole that allows the pancreas to drain into the duodenum)
- Most patient gets complete relief from pancreatitis after MPS
- The treatment is considered very safe
- Many doctors also insert a stent into the minor papilla after the cut is made

- The stent is a short tube that keeps the papilla open so the pancreas can drain
- It is a short-term fix (the stent should fall out within1 week so it doesn't become clogged)
- If the stent doesn't fall out on its own, it needs to be removed (using an endoscope)

10. WHAT IS THE PROGNOSIS

10.1 Looking Toward the Long-Term

The prognosis (long-term outlook) for those with pancreatitis is generally good. However, the prognosis depends on a number of variables including the number and severity of attacks, whether the pancreatitis is acute or chronic (including hereditary), how much damage has been done to the pancreas and other organs, and the extent of malnutrition, if any.

Usually, people with acute pancreatitis experience complete recovery.

- If the cause—such as gallstones—is removed, pancreatitis likely will not recur
- If the cause is unable to be removed or rectified—such as in pancreas divisum—diet and lifestyle changes can have a dramatic and positive impact on the prognosis
- If the cause is unknown (i.e., idiopathic), additional diagnostic testing may be needed until a cause is identified

In chronic (and hereditary) pancreatitis, the prognosis is also generally good. However, this is dependent upon dietary and lifestyle changes and taking medications exactly as prescribed.

With any type of pancreatitis, it is absolutely necessary to stop smoking and avoid alcoholic beverages entirely. Alcohol can contribute to inflammation of and damage to the pancreas, while smoking stresses the body's defenses against inflammation.

11. A FEW RELIABLE RESOURCES

11.1 American Gastroenterological Associa

"The American Gastroenterological Association is the trusted voice of the GI community. Founded in 1897, the AGA has grown to include 17,000 members from around the globe who are involved in all aspects of the science, practice and advancement of gastroenterology. The AGA Institute administers the practice, research and educational programs of the organization."

http://www.gastro.org/patient-center

http://www.gastro.org/patient-center/digestive-conditions/pancreatitis

11.2 Johns Hopkins Medicine Gastroenterology and Hepatology

"U.S. News & World Report has ranked the Johns Hopkins Hospital as the #1 hospital for the past 19 consecutive years."

http://www.hopkins-gi.org/

11.3 Mayo Clinic

"Mayo Clinic is a not-for-profit medical practice dedicated to the diagnosis and treatment of virtually every type of complex illness."

"More than 3,300 physicians, scientists and researchers from Mayo Clinic share their expertise to empower you to manage your health."

"Since 1904, millions of people from all walks of life have found answers at Mayo Clinic."

http://www.mayoclinic.com/health/pancreatitis/DS00371

11.4 Merck Manual of Diagnosis and Therapy for HealthCare Professionals

"Merck is committed to bringing out the best in medicine. As part of that effort, Merck has created *The Merck Manuals*, a series of healthcare books for medical professionals and consumers. As a service to the community, the content of *The Manuals* is now available in enhanced online versions as part of *The Merck Manuals Online Medical Library*. The Online Medical Library is updated periodically with new information, and contains photographs, and audio and video material not present in the print versions."

http://www.merck.com/mmpe/sec02/ch015/ch015a.html

11.5 National Institutes of Health (NIH)

The NIH is "one of the world's foremost medical research centers and the federal focal point for medical research in the United States." (Parker 9)

- National Library of Medicine:
  http://www.nlm.nih.gov/medlineplus/healthtopics.html

- National Institute of Diabetes and Digestive and Kidney Diseases:
  http://www2.niddk.nih.gov/HealthEducation/default

- National Digestive Diseases Information Clearinghouse (NDDIC):
  http://digestive.niddk.nih.gov/ddiseases/pubs/pancreatitis

11.6 Science Daily

"ScienceDaily is one of the Internet's most popular science news web sites. Since starting in 1995, the award-winning site has earned the loyalty of students, researchers, healthcare professionals, government agencies, educators and the general public around the world. Now with more than 3 million monthly visitors, ScienceDaily generates nearly 15 million page views a month and is steadily growing in its global audience."

http://www.ScienceDaily.com

11.7 University of Cincinnati Pancreatic Disease Center

"Our mission of The UC Pancreatic Disease Center is to deliver outstanding, compassionate care to patients with pancreatic tumors and pancreatitis. We strive to improve the lives of our patients through innovative clinical and basic research in pancreatic disease."

"With national recognition for treatments of pancreatitis and pancreatic cancer, many patients travel from all over the United States. Our physicians, nurses, and staff have been awarded honors in outstanding patient care, year after year."

"The UC Pancreatic Disease Center is located in Cincinnati, Ohio; in the heart of the University of Cincinnati campus."

http://www.ucpancreas.org/pancreatitis.htm

11.8 WebMD

"WebMD provides valuable health information, tools for managing your health, and support to those who seek information. You can trust that our content is timely and credible."

"The WebMD content staff blends award-winning expertise in medicine, journalism, health communication and content creation to bring you the best health information possible. Our esteemed colleagues at MedicineNet.com are frequent contributors to WebMD and comprise our Medical Editorial Board. Our Independent Medical Review Board continuously reviews the site for accuracy and timeliness."

http://www.webmd.com/digestive-disorders/digestive-diseases-pancreatitis

11.9 Print Journals

In addition, there are a number of major journals that discuss pancreatitis and related conditions and diseases:

The Journal of the American Medical Association (JAMA)
www.jama.ama-assn.org/

The New England Journal of Medicine's Gastroenterology Collection
http://content.nejm.org/cgi/collection/gastroenterology

Gastroenterology: Official Journal of the American Gastroenterological Association
http://www.gastrojournal.org/

12. EATING FOR PANCREATITIS

First, let me give an introduction to some dietary terminology, from the USDA's website (http://www.nal.usda.gov/fnic/dga/dga95/lowfat.html).

- Fat-free = 0.5 grams (or, ½ gram) or less of fat in one serving of a food item
- Low-fat = 3 grams or less of fat in one serving of a food item
- Reduced fat = a food item which is at least 25% fat
- Light = one-third (1/3) fewer calories and/or 50% less fat

Also, when it comes to describing liquids…

- Clear fluid or liquid = you can see through it
- Colorless fluid or liquid = has no color
- For example:
  - Apple juice is clear but not colorless
  - Water is clear AND colorless

One of the most important nutritional concepts to keep in mind—and this is true for just about anyone, but especially those with pancreatitis—is to drink a lot of liquids. Liquids can be water, fruit juice, milk (low-fat or fat-free/skim), soups and broths, tea, decaffeinated coffee, and so on. Dehydration, or a lack of sufficient fluid in the body, can increase the likelihood or worsen attacks of pancreatitis.

Also, keep in mind that vegetables and fruits have a very high water content—that is, they are mostly water. If you have pancreatitis and you've read this guidebook, then you know, by now, that your pancreas is already damaged. And, if your pancreas is already damaged, then anything you throw at it will just serve for further stress it, and possibly even damage it more. Soft and liquid foods, and foods that are largely water (like fruits) do not put as much strain on the pancreas as solid, tough-to-digest foods, like steak or beef, and fats.

Another very important nutritional concept is calories, or how much food you eat. It is highly recommended that you work with a nutritionist or registered dietitian to determine the correct amount of calories for you. Excess weight (due to excess calories, lack of exercise, and so on) can also increase the likelihood or worsen attacks of pancreatitis. Excess fat in the body produces chemicals (actually, proteins) called *cytokines*. Cytokines, in turn, cause inflammation throughout the body—and we know what inflammation of the pancreas is.

The third very important nutritional concept is fat itself—and by this I mean fat consumption, from the foods you eat. Fat is high in calories, so it can worsen weight gain or hinder weight loss. Fat is also difficult to digest and can cause additional strain on the pancreas, especially if your acinar cells are damaged (remember, those are the cells that produce the fat-digesting enzymes). Avoid fat—all oils, butter, margarine, lard, and so on. You can discuss with your doctor the advantages and disadvantages of fish oil. If you have difficulty digesting oil (which is liquid fat), then you probably need to avoid all oils—including fish oil.

You will need to check the ingredients of all the foods you purchase. You will likely be stunned by the number of food products that are made with oil! Oil is everywhere and in just about every processed food item, especially anything snack-like, and even fajita shells and wraps. Even most pretzels are made with oil or butter, though there are a few fat-free pretzel options.

The last major nutritional concept to keep in mi,
every meal and snack should contain both carbo,
and protein. As a matter of fact, ideally, every m(
snack should contain protein, fat, and carbohydrates (
but you really do need to watch the fat content.

In terms of protein, most dietitians and diet-type books
recommend 2 servings of protein per meal and 1 serving of
protein per snack. A serving of protein is about 7 or 8
grams of protein—I'm sure you can do the math.

You'll need to check with your doctor and a nutritionist or
registered dietitian, though, for your own specifics. The
amount of carbs and protein your body can handle depends
on a number of factors including diabetes, kidney
disease/damage, and so on.

Foods to Consider

These lists are neither extensive nor exhaustive, but they
will give you a good idea of the range of low-fat or non-fat
foods available for you to eat.

Fruits

- Apples & applesauce
- Bananas
- Grapes
- Oranges & orange juice
- Peach
- Pumpkin
- Strawberries
- Watermelon
- And many others

Vegetables

- Broccoli
- Broccoli rabe (aka, broccoli rapini)
- Carrots
- Cauliflower
- Celery
- Corn and corn on the cob
- Cucumber
- Escarole
- Lettuce
- Onion
- Peas
- Pepper (bell; hot; sweet; cherry; etc…)
- Spaghetti squash
- Spinach
- Tomato
- Yam
- Zucchini / Yellow Squash
- And many others

Bread and Other Starches

- Bread, multigrain
- Bread, pita
- Bread, rye
- Rice, brown
- English muffin (light or whole grain)
- Fig bars, fat free (e.g., fat-free Fig Newtons)
- Pasta
- Oatmeal, 1-minute (instant) or old fashioned (which takes longer to cook)

Protein

- Beans, Cannellini (or, white)
- Beans, Ceci (chickpeas or garbanzo beans)
- Beans, Lupini (common in Italian delis or markets)
- Beans, Kidney (red)
- Beans, Refried (Old El Pasto Traditional refried beans is very low in fat, 0.5 grams per serving; most refried beans are _not_ low fat)
- Canadian bacon, lean
- Chicken breast (in limited amounts due to its fat content)
- Cream Cheese, Fat Free
- Egg substitute
- Egg whites
- Ham, extra lean or 90% fat free
- Lobster Delights (Alaskan Pollock)
- Milk, skim (e.g., fat free Over the Moon milk has extra milk protein and tastes like 2% reduced fat milk)
- Orange roughy
- Shrimp
- Turkey breast (without the skin; also in limited amounts due to its fat content)
- Yogurt (non-fat or low-fat; check the label)

A Sample Meal Plan

Here's a simplified example of a very low-fat meal plan:

Breakfast	1 cup orange juice ½ cup egg whites + 1 slice deli ham or Canadian bacon + ¼ cup bell pepper & onion 1 whole grain English muffin with fat-free cream cheese Coffee with fat-free milk
Snack	Fat-free cream cheese and celery 1 piece or serving of fruit Water
Lunch	Deli ham & sliced tomato on whole grain bread OR Shrimp with cocktail sauce 1 piece or serving of fruit 2 fat-free Fig Newtons or 1 serving of baby carrots Water
Snack	Banana and strawberry smoothie Or Egg whites + 1 slice deli ham on whole grain English muffin
Dinner	2 – 3 servings of chicken, turkey, ham, or pork Salad with fat-free (or no) dressing Plain cooked pasta, potato, or rice Homemade unsweetened iced tea
Snack	Fat-free pudding

Meal Planning as Easy as P-F-C

It is important to ensure that every meal and snack is composed of at least one serving of protein (P), (ideally) a little bit of fat (F), and some carbohydrate (C), for the following reasons:

- To satisfy your hunger
- To maintain steady or even blood sugar levels [so you don't overeat later]
- To reduce the risk of muscle loss from inadequate protein,.

The problem with pancreatitis sufferers is, obviously, the fat, so in many cases, your snacks and meals may contain no fat at all, and that's okay.

Here are some examples of meals and snacks using the P-F-C philosophy. Again, run this past your doctor to ensure it is appropriate for you based on your overall health and any other medical conditions you may have.

Breakfast

- Egg white (P), low-fat cheese(PF), and vegetable (C) omelet with orange juice (C) and a slice of whole wheat toast (C)
- Oatmeal (PFC) with fat-free milk (PC)
- Low-fat (F) yogurt (PC)

Lunch

- Salad with veggies (C); beans (P) & cheese (P); fruit (C)
- Shrimp cocktail (P) + apple crisp (FC)

Dinner

- Escarole (C) and bean (P) soup with chicken (PF) and 2 slices of Italian bread (C)
- Refried beans (PF) with low-fat cheese (PF), taco sauce (C), salsa (C), corn (C)
- Minestrone or vegetable soup (PFC)
- Pasta (PC) with shrimp (P) and tomato sauce (C)
- Pasta e fagioli (PFC), or pasta and bean soup
- Steamed shrimp (P) and vegetables (C) over rice(C)
- Grilled chicken (PC) with grilled vegetables (C) and a side of fruit (C)

Snacks

- Apple crisp: apples (C), oatmeal (PFC), cinnamon, applesauce (C)
- Celery with fat-free cream cheese (P) and a side of fruit (C)
- Egg whites (P), a slice of ham (PF) on a whole grain English muffin (C)
- Low-fat string cheese (PF) and fat-free pretzels (C)
- Pumpernickel or rye bagel (C) with fat-free cream cheese (P)

A SAMPLING OF LOW-FAT OR FAT-FREE RECIPES FOR PANCREATITIS

- Apple Cake
- Apple Crisp
- Apples, Cooked
- Carrot Cake, Low-Fat Super-Moist
- Chicken & Pasta with Peppers, Spinach/broccoli rabe, & Garlic
- Fish, Parmesan-Crusted
- Omelet, Egg-White
- Salad, Mexi-Mix
- Salad, Simple
- Shrimp & Pasta
- Smoothie
- Soup, Mediterranean Chicken

Apple Cake

Ingredients

5	Large red delicious apples
1 cup	Applesauce
1 cup	Egg substitute
1 cup	Organic brown sugar
½ cup	White (granulated) sugar
2 tsp	Cinnamon
2 cups	Flour

Preparation Steps

1. Preheat oven to 350°F
2. Lightly coat 13 x 9 x 2 ½ inch baking dish with non-stick cooking spray
3. In a large mixing bowl, mix together applesauce, egg substitute, sugars, cinnamon, and flour
4. Peel, core, and cut the apples into bite-sized pieces
5. Place the apples in the baking dish
6. Pour batter on top of the apples and spread out evenly (as much as is possible!)
7. Bake for 45 to 55 minutes

APPLE CRISP

Ingredients

5 or 6	red delicious apples
1 ½ cups	oatmeal (instant or 1-minute works best, but old fashioned works also)
3 Tbsp	cinnamon
1 ½ cups	applesauce

Preparation Steps

1. Spray a glass loaf pan with non-stick cooking spray
2. Preheat over to 325 degrees Fahrenheit
3. Pour orange juice into loaf pan
4. Cut apples into bite-sized pieces
5. Sprinkle with 1 to 2 Tbsp of cinnamon
6. Mix thoroughly
7. In a separate bowl, mix oatmeal, remaining cinnamon, and apple sauce thoroughly
8. Spread oatmeal mixture over apples and smooth to a flat surface
9. Place loaf pan in over and cook (uncovered) for 55 minutes

APPLES, COOKED

Ingredients

6	Red delicious apples—peeled & diced
¾ cup	Orange juice (no pulp)
1 ½ tsp	Cinnamon

Preparation Steps

1. Spray a medium sized pot with non-stick cooking spray
2. Add orange juice
3. Turn heat to medium
4. Add apples
5. Add cinnamon
6. Stir thoroughly
7. Cover with a lid
8. Cook until apples are tender—but, stir frequently so the apples don't stick or burn

CARROT CAKE, LOW-FAT SUPER-MOIST

- 1 cup organic brown sugar
- 2 cupsall purpose flour
- 1 tsp baking powder
- 1 tsp baking soda
- 1 tsp salt
- 1 tsp cinnamon
- 3 cupsfinely shredded carrots
- 2 cups natural (unsweetened) apple sauce
- Egg substitute equivalent to 4 large eggs
- 2 tsp vanilla

1. In a large mixing bowl, combine first 7 ingredients.
2. Add carrots, applesauce, eggs, vanilla
3. Beat for 2 to 3 minutes on medium
4. Pour into greased and floured 9x13 inch pan
5. Bake in oven at 325 F for 45 minutes
6. Cool on rack
7. Frost with cream cheese frosting & refrigerate

Cream Cheese Frosting

- 3 oz of low-fat (or fat free) cream cheese (softened)
- ¼ cup butter (softened)
- 1 tsp vanilla
- 1 ½ cups confectioners sugar

1. In large mixing bowl, beat together cream cheese, butter, and vanilla until light and fluffy.
2. Gradually add confectioners sugar and beat until smooth
3. Spread over cooled cake.

CHICKEN & PASTA WITH PEPPERS, SPINACH/BROCCOLI RABE, & GARLIC

- 2 pounds   Organic chicken breast meat
- 1 bag   Baby spinach or broccoli rabe/rapini
- 3 cloves   garlic, fresh or jarred in water
- 1 ½ cups   roasted red peppers (jarred, in water)
- 1 cup   chicken broth (or water)
- ½ pound   small pasta (ziti, penne, etc…)
- ¼ cup   fresh, grated cheese

Preparation Steps

1. Prepare the pasta as directed on the box
2. Cut the chicken into bite-size pieces
3. Cook chicken over medium-low heat in frying pan with non-stick cooking spray until just thoroughly cooked (stir frequently!)
4. In a medium saucepan or small pot, coat with a thin layer of non-stick cooking spray
5. Turn on the heat to medium-high
6. Add the chicken broth
7. Add the spinach, diced or thinly sliced garlic, and roasted red peppers
8. Add a pinch or two of salt and some black pepper
9. Cook over medium-high heat until the spinach is very wilted
10. Add ¼ cup grated cheese (parmesan or romano)
11. Mix well
12. When pasta is finished, drain thoroughly
13. Place pasta, chicken, and spinach or broccoli rabe mixture into the frying pat or large pot
14. Mix thoroughly, then serve

FISH, PARMESAN-CRUSTED

Ingredients

12 oz	Alaskan Pollock (or any mild fish)
¾ Cup	Freshly grated Parmesan cheese
1 whole	Egg
	Black pepper
	Onion powder

Preparation Steps

1. Preheat oven to 350 degrees Fahrenheit
2. Lightly coat a small baking pan with non-stick cooking spray
3. Thoroughly beat 1 egg in a bowl
4. In a separate bowl, combine the cheese, black pepper, and onion powder—stir together with a fork or spoon a few times to mix the ingredients together
5. Cut the fish into palm-sized pieces
6. Dip the fish in the egg, coating the fish on all sides
7. Dip the egg-coated fish into the cheese mixture—try to get the cheese mixture all around the fish (it won't be coated in cheese but that's OK)
8. Place the cheese-coated fish on the pan
9. Bake in the oven for 15 minutes

Serve with a side of fresh (or frozen) vegetables and maybe a small piece of bread (like sourdough, rye, pumpernickel or even ciabatta)

<u>O</u>MELET, <u>E</u>GG-<u>W</u>HITE

- 1 cup egg whites (I use the kind that comes in a carton)
- ¼ cup diced bell pepper (green, yellow, red, orange, whatever)
- ¼ cup diced onion
- ¼ cup diced zucchini
- 1 to 2 oz low-fat ham (if you prefer some meat)
- non-stick cooking spray (I prefer the canola oil variety)

1. Coat a small frying pan lightly with non-stick cooking spray
2. Turn on heat to medium low
3. Put ham and all the vegetables into the pan
4. Simmer for about 2 minutes while sliding everything around so it doesn't stick
5. Spray the pan and vegetables with non-stick spray again
6. Pour the egg whites into the pan
7. Stir occasionally so the egg whites don't stick
8. Serve with a side of whole or cut fruit or a slice of whole grain/rye/pumpernickel bread and a glass of real fruit juice

SALAD, MEXI-MIX

Ingredients

½ cup	Corn
1 cup	White rice
8 oz	Refried beans*
1 oz	Low-fat or fat-free cheese, shredded
½	Tomato (fresh, raw)
3 Tbsp	Salsa
1 cup	Shredded lettuce
3 Tbsp	Taco sauce
½	Onion (fresh, raw)
½	Bell pepper (fresh, raw)

* Old El Paso Traditional are very low fat

Preparation Steps

1. Spray a small pot or frying pan with non-stick cooking spray
2. Add water to about ¼ inch deep into the pan/pot
3. Add onion and bell pepper
4. Put lid on pot/pan
5. Cook on medium until tender
6. Meanwhile, cook the rice (I use instant rice in a bag that cooks in 10 minutes in a microwave)
7. When the rice is finished, cook the corn (I microwave frozen corn in water for about 6 minutes)
8. Once the onions and peppers are cooked, drain the pan/pot of any excess water and remove the peppers and onions to a bowl
9. Turn the heat to medium-low

10. Spray the pot or pan again with non-stick cooking spray
11. Pour the refried beans into the pot or pan and heat through (about 5 to 7 minutes or so)—stir frequently so they don't stick and burn
12. Once the beans are finished, turn off the heat
13. Spoon the rice onto a place
14. Spoon the beans onto the rice
15. Sprinkle the beans with the shredded cheese
16. Put onions and peppers on top of cheese
17. Put the corn on top
18. Add the remaining ingredients (lettuce, tomato, salsa, taco sauce) and enjoy

SALAD, SIMPLE

- 1 ½ cups of lettuce (romaine, iceberg, spring mix, or whatever you like)
- 6 baby carrots
- ¼ cup onion (raw)
- ½ cup bell pepper (red, green, orange, yellow)
- ½ stalk celery
- 5 to 6 oz beans, canned (Lupini; red kidney; white cannellini; etc…)
- ¼ cucumber (with or without skin, your choice)
- 2 oz fat-free or low-fat cheese
- Salt, to taste
- Pepper (black or cracked), to taste
- Oregano, to taste
- Onion powder, to taste
- 2 to 3 Tbsp Fat-free salad dressing (or, use a couple dashes of vinegar)

Preparation Steps

1. Thoroughly cleanse all vegetables (carrots, onion, lettuce, bell pepper, celery, cucumber)
2. Rinse the beans under running water
3. Using a clean, unused paper towel, dry the vegetables until only slightly moist
4. Put all vegetables into a bowl
5. Put on the salad dressing
6. Add a dash each (to your taste or liking) of black pepper, sea salt, oregano, onion powder, or other spices and herbs, if you prefer
7. Top with the cheese (alternately, you can sprinkle on grated cheese, like you would for pasta; fresh grated cheese is best!)

SHRIMP & PASTA

Ingredients

1 cup	Pasta (cooked)
10 jumbo	Shrimp (cleaned & deveined)
½ cup	Tomato sauce
1 to 2 Tbsp	Grated cheese (Romano, Parmesan)

Preparation Steps

1. Boil the shrimp until they are firm but still tender
2. At the same time, prepare the pasta using the directions on the pasta box
3. Prepare the tomato sauce (your own, or canned/jarred)
4. When the shrimp & pasta are each finished cooking, drain thoroughly
5. Pour the pasta into a serving bowl
6. Top the pasta with the tomato sauce and grated cheese
7. Mix in the shrimp

This is somewhat of a bland recipe, but certainly very low in fat. To spice it up, you can add sliced hot peppers (or jarred hot pepper seeds); you can also add sautéed spinach (sautee it in a little bit of cooking spray and water with some diced fresh garlic). Adding fresh basil to the recipe adds additional flavor as well.

SMOOTHIE

- 1 whole, very ripe banana
- 4 large strawberries (or 6 small ones)
- 6oz container of Weight Watchers yogurt (for example, the peach yogurt has 0.5 grams fat per 6oz serving
- ¼ cup orange juice
- 5 whole ice cubes

Preparation Steps

1. Place all the ingredients in a blender
2. Blend until smooth and creamy
3. Pour into a glass and serve (I like to drink mine with a straw)

Note: if you use vanilla or even plain yogurt, you may need to add 1 to 1 ½ tablespoons of sugar or an artificial sweetener, if you prefer your smoothie on the sweeter side

Also, these ingredients usually give about 2 full cups of smoothie—enough for 2 separate servings. I store the extra in the refrigerator—it stays for at least a couple of days. I've even prepared this in the evening and taken it to work the next day in a spill-proof container.

SOUP, MEDITERRANEAN CHICKEN

- 32 oz chicken broth (I use organic, fat free)
- 2 cups water (spring, purified, or filtered)
- 2 cups baby spinach (fresh, raw)
- 15 to 16 oz can red or white (kidney or cannellini) beans
- 1 whole onion
- 1 stalk celery
- 8 baby carrots
- 29 oz can tomato sauce (I use Hunt's plain; it's unseasoned)
- ½ lb (8 oz) small pasta, uncooked (pastina or orzo or acini de pepe)
- 12.5 oz can chicken (white meat only, in water)
- 1/3 cup grated cheese (like Romano)
- ¼ tsp black pepper
- ½ tsp onion powder

Preparation Steps

1. Pour chicken broth and 1 cup (8 oz) water into a large pot
2. Turn heat to high
3. Dice celery, onion, and carrot and add to broth
4. Bring broth to a boil
5. Boil for 15 minutes (until veggies are tender)
6. Add baby spinach and beans & chicken, black pepper, onion powder
7. Add another 8 oz (1 cup) water
8. Add tomato sauce
9. Bring to a boil
10. Add pasta
11. Bring to a boil (stir frequently)

12. Boil until pasta is just done (stir frequently so pasta doesn't stick to the pot)
13. Turn off heat
14. Add cheese and stir thoroughly

You can store leftover soup, covered, in the refrigerator for about 2 or 3 days (the chicken will eventually go bad).

REFERENCES

"Acute Pancreatitis." (2010)
<http://enotes.tripod.com/pancreatitis.htm>.

"Antioxidants Offer Pain Relief In Patients With Chronic
Pancreatitis." American Gastroenterological
Association. (11 January11 2009)
<http://www.sciencedaily.com
/releases/2009/01/090101083304.htm>.

"Autoimmune Pancreatitis." The Mayo Clinic. (17 July
2010) <http://www.mayoclinic.org/autoimmune-
pancreatitis/>.

"Calorie Restricted Diet Prevents Pancreatic Inflammation
And Cancer, Study Suggests." University of Texas
M. D. Anderson Cancer Center. (17 April 2008)
<http://www.sciencedaily.com/releases/2008/04/08
0414171502.htm>.

"Chronic Pancreatitis." University of Cincinnati.
<http://www.ucpancreas.org/chronicpancreatitis.ht
m>.

"Creon." RxList, Inc. (28 April 2010)
<http://www.rxlist.com/creon-drug.htm>

"Does Hypertriglyceridemia Aggravate Episodes Of Severe
Acute Pancreatitis?" World Journal of
Gastroenterology 13 October 2008
<http://www.sciencedaily.com
/releases/2008/10/081014114850.htm>

"Hereditary Pancreatitis" University of Cincinnati.
<http://www.ucpancreas.org/hereditarypancreatitis.
htm>.

"High Triglyceride Levels Common, Often Untreated
Among Americans." JAMA and Archives Journals.
(30 March 2009)

<http://www.sciencedaily.com/releases/2009/03/09
0323161117.htm>.

"Hypotension, Low Blood Pressure." Homeopathy for
Everyone (4 June 2009)
<http://health.hpathy.com/blood-low-pressure-
symptoms-treatment.asp>.

"Lipoic Acid Found to Reduce Triglycerides by 60 Percent
in Lab Rats." (18 November 2009)
<http://seniorjournal.com/news/nutrition-
vitamins/2009/20090401-lipoicacidfound.htm>.

"New approach discovered to lowering triglycerides." (18
November 2009)
<http://www.eurekalert.org/pub_releases/2009-
03/osu-nad033009.php>.

"Pancreas." Encyclopedia Britannica Online. (16 July
2010)
<http://www.britannica.com/EBchecked/topic-
art/275485/68636/Structures-of-the-pancreas-
Acinar-cells-produce-digestive-enzymes-which>.

"Pancreas: Function." University of Montana (16 July
2010)
<http://www.montana.edu/wwwai/lmsd/alcohol/van
essa/vwpancreas.htm>.

"Pancreatitis." University of Cincinnati.
<http://www.ucpancreas.org/pancreatitis.htm>.

"Pancreatitis." Mayo Clinic. (17 January 2009)
<http://www.mayoclinic.com/health/pancreatitis/DS
00371>.

"Pancreatitis." National Digestive Diseases Information
Clearinghouse, NIH Publication No. 08–1596 (July
2008)
<http://digestive.niddk.nih.gov/ddiseases/pubs/panc
reatitis>.

"Pancreatitis." The Merck Manual for Healthcare Professionals. (2010) Merck Sharp and Dohme Corporation. <http://www.merck.com/mmpe/sec02/ch015/ch015 a.html>.

"Pancreatitis." University of Montana (16 July 2010) <http://www.montana.edu/wwwai/imsd/alcohol/Va nessa/vwpancreas.htm>.

"Popular Diabetes Treatment Could Trigger Pancreatitis, Pancreatic Cancer, Study Suggests." University of California—Los Angeles. (1 May 2009) <http://www.sciencedaily.com /releases/2009/04/090430161238.htm>.

"Study Redefines Roles Of Alcohol, Smoking In Risk For Pancreatitis." JAMA and Archives Journals. (11 June 2009) <http://www.sciencedaily.com/releases/2009/06/09 0608162430.htm>.

"Tips to Remember: Anaphylaxis." American Academy of Allergy, Asthma & Immunology. (2010) <http://www.aaaai.org/patients/publicedmat/tips/wh atisanaphylaxis.stm>.

"Why Alcohol Is Bad For Your Pancreas." Journal of Clinical Investigation. (9 June 2008). <http://www.sciencedaily.com/releases/2008/06/08 0605203902.htm>.

Basturk, MD, Olca and Ipek Coban MD, and Volkan Adsay MD. "Pancreatic Cysts: Pathologic Classification, Differential Diagnosis, and Clinical Implications." Archives of Pathologic Laboratory Medicine 133 (March 2009):423-439.

Czako, Laslo. "Diagnosis of early-stage chronic pancreatitis by secretin-enhanced magnetic

resonance cholangiopancreatopgrahy." Journal of
Gastroenterology 42[Suppl XVII](2007):133-117

De Filippo, Massimo and Emiliano Giudici, Nicola
Sverzellati, Maurizio Zompatori. "Pancreas divisum
and duodenal diverticula as two causes of acute or
chronic pancreatitis that should not be overlooked:
a case report." Journal of Medical Case Reports
2:166 (19 May 2008).

DiMagno, Matthew J. and Eugene P. DiMagno. "Chronic
Pancreatitis." Current Opinion in Gastroenterology.
25.5 (2009):454-459.

Dugdale III, MD, David and George F. Longstreth, MD.
"Pancreatitis." National Institutes of Health (2008
November 17)
<http://www.nlm.nih.gov/medlineplus/ency/article/
001144.htm>.

Freedman, MD, PhD, Steven D. "Acute Pancreatitis."
Merck Manuals Online Medical Library (2007) 16
July 2010
<http://www.merck.com/mmpe/print/sec02/ch015/c
h015b.html>.

Ghattas Khoury, MD, Ghattas and Samer S. Deeba MD.
"Pancreatitis." (26 Jan 2009)
<http://emedicine.medscape.com/article/775867-
overview>.

Hammond, Bethanie and Gary C. Vitale MD, Nick
Rangnekar MD, Emily A. Vitale, John C. Binford.
"Bilateral Thorascopic Splanchnicectomy for Pain
Control in Chronic Pancreatitis." The American
Surgeon 70.6(June 2007):546-549.

Kamisawa, MD, PhD, Terumi. "Is there a causal
relationship between pancreas divisum and

pancreatic cancer?" Journal of Gastroenterology 41 (2006):1131-1132.

Kashyap, Ajit Singh; Anand, Kuldip Parkash; Kashyap, Surekha. "Severe Acute Pancreatitis." JAMA: Journal of the American Medical Association 292.11(15 September 2004):1305.

Kwan, Vu and Sze M. Loh, Patrick R. Walsh, Stephen J. Williams, Michael J. Bourke. "Minor Papilla Sphincterotomy for Pancreatitis Due to Pancreas Divisum." ANZ Journal of Surgery 78 (2008):257-261.

Lee, Julia and Wan Ip, Peter Durie. 'Is fibrosing colonopathy an immune mediated disease?" Archives of Disease in Childhood 77 (1997):66-70.

Löhr, J. Matthias. What are the useful biological and functional markers of early-stage chronic pancreatitis? Journal of Gastroenterology 2007; 42[Suppl XVII]:66-71.

Mine, MD, PhD, Tetusya. Is post-endoscopic retrograde cholangiopancreatography pancreatitis the same as acute clinical pancreatitis? Journal of Gastroenterology 2007: 42:265-266.

Mortelé, MD, Koenraa J. and Tatiana C. Rocha, MD, Jonathan L. Streeter, MD, Andrew J. Taylor, MD. "Multimodal Imaging of Pancreatic and Biliary Congential Anomalies." RadioGraphics: The Journal of Continuing Medical Education in Radiology. 26 (May 2006):715-731. <http://radiographics.rsna.org/content/26/3/715.full>.

Multimodality Imaging of Pancreatic and Biliary Congenital Anomalies. May 2006 RadioGraphics, 26, 715-731.

Munoz, MD, Abilio and David A Katerndahl, MD.
"Diagnosis and Management of Acute Pancreatitis."
American Academy of Family Physicians. (July
2010)
<http://www.aafp.org/afp/20000701/164.html>.

Ng, Wendy K. and Osman Tarabain MD. Pancreas
divisum: a cause of idiopathic acute pancreatitis.
CMAJ, April 28, 2009: 180(9): 949-951 – by

Nishino, Takayoshi and Fumitake Toki, Itaru Ot, Hiroyasu
Oyama, Takashi Hatori, Keiko Shiratori.Prevalence
of pancreatic and biliary tract tumors in pancreas
divisum.   Journal of Gastroenterology 2006;
41:1088-1093.

Parker, MD, James N. and Philip M. Parker, MD. The
Official Patient's Sourcebook on Pancreatitis. 2002
ICON Group International, Inc.

Prognosis and Prognostic Factors In Chronic Pancreatitis.
JAMA: Journal of the American Medical
Association. 9/1/89, 262(9), 1238

Richards, CCN, Byron. "R-Alpha Lipoic Acid Lowers
Triglycerides." (18 November 2009)
<http://www.wellnessresources.com/main/printable/
r-alpha_lipoic_acid_lowers_triglycerides>.

Sahelian, MD, Ray. "Pancreatitis natural treatment,
vitamins herbs supplements and antioxidants." (5
July 2010)
<http://www.raysahelian.com/pancreatitis.html>.

Schnelldorfer, MD, Thomas and David B. Adams, MD.
Surgical Treatment of Alcohol-Associated Chronic
Pancreatitis: The Challenges and Pitfalls. Pages
503-509 The American Surgeon vol 74 #6 june
2008.

Schnelldorfer, MD, Thomas and David B. Adams, MD.
The Effect of Malnutrition on Morbidity After
Surgery for Chronic Pancreatitis. By pages 466-473
The American Surgeon june 2005 vol 71 # 6

Spicak, Julius and Petra Poulova, Jitka Plucnarova, Marek
Rehor, Helena Filipova, Tomas Hucl. Pancreas
divisum does not modify the natural course of
chronic pancreatitis. By – Journal of
Gastroenterology 2007; 42:135-139

Sugiyama, Masanori and Hiroki Haradome, and Yutaka
Atomi. Magnetic resonance imaging for diagnosing
chronic pancreatitis. Journal of Gastroenterology
2007; 42[Suppl XVII]:108-112.

Torpy, Janet M. (2008 April 2). Pancreatitis. JAMA:
Journal of the American Medical Association,
299(13), 1630.

Vertebral Osteonecrosis Associated with Pancreatitis in a
Woman with Pancreas Divisum. Freyr G.
Sigmundsson, Peter B. Andersen MD, Henrik D.
Schroeder MD DMSc, Karsten Thomsen, MD
DMSc. The Journal of Bone and Joint Surgery.
Vol 86-A, #11, 11/2004.

Vitale, MD, Gary C. and Brian R Davis MD, Carlos
Zavaleta MD, Michael Vitale MD, James K
Fullerton, MD.Endoscopic Retrograde
Cholangiopancreatography and Histopathology
Correlation for Chronic Pancreatitis. The
American Surgeon. Aug 2009, vol 75 #8 pp 649-
653.

Made in the USA
Middletown, DE
10 December 2017